CONTEN

INTRODUCTION

No matter what your age, or what your state of physical health might be, exercise is absolutely essential to maintaining and improving both your physical and mental well-being. This does not mean that you have to join a gym or hire a personal trainer. The fact is that there are many easy ways to get your body moving and improve your health – even if you are housebound!

Some of the reasons why seniors do not follow an exercise program includes: concerns about injury or falls; not knowing where to begin; ongoing health problems or disabilities; or feeling you are too old or too frail. These concerns need not stop you.

I have designed a series of exercises you can do whether you are confined to your house, or even to your bed. These exercises will help you stay strong and energetic, help manage the symptoms of illness and pain, and even reverse some of the symptoms of aging. Exercise is also good for your mind, elevating mood and improving memory. No matter what your age or current physical condition, you can benefit from exercise.

This book is intended to take you step by step through a program of exercises, with illustrations to help you assure you are doing them safely and correctly. Let's get going!

DISCLAIMER

STOP!

BEFORE STARTING THIS OR ANY OTHER EXERCISE PROGRAM, CONSULT YOUR PHYSICIAN.

The information provided in this book is designed to provide helpful information on the subjects discussed. This book is not meant to be used, nor should it be used, to diagnose or treat any medical condition. For diagnosis or treatment of any medical problem, consult your own physician. The publisher Easy in Fitness and author Neville Warburton are not responsible for any specific health or allergy needs that may require medical supervision and are not liable for any damages or negative consequences from any treatment, action, application or preparation, to any person reading or following the information in this book. References are provided for informational purposes only and do not constitute endorsement of any websites or other sources.

Chest

Lie on your back with your legs 6 to 8 inches apart with toes towards the ceiling

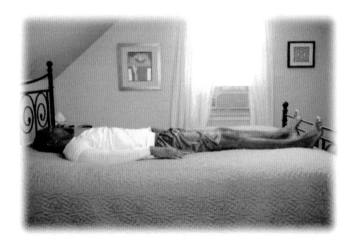

Have your arms straight; lock your elbows, with your palms up

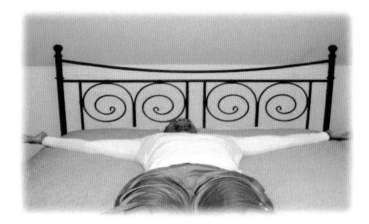

With arms straight put fingertips together in front of you and press

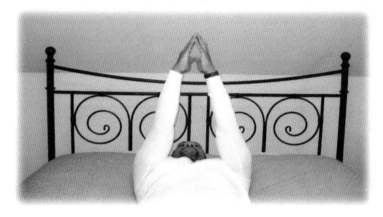

Hold for two (2) seconds
Then return arms to the bed, palms up and fingers apart

Arms straight press arms into bed

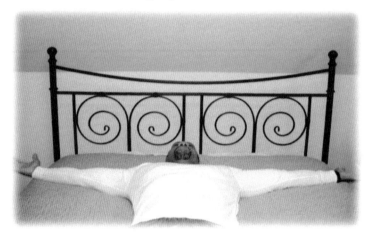

Hold for two (2) seconds
Repeat six (6) times

Anterior Deltoids

Lie on your right side with your head rested on your right arm, legs together

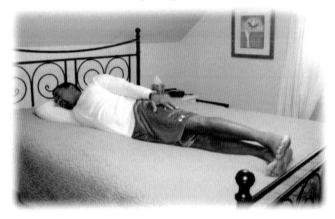

Raise left arm straight, lock elbow palm facing forward with fingers apart

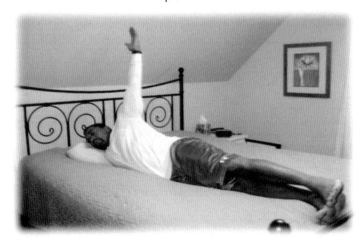

While keeping arm straight reach back
Hold for two (2) seconds
Repeat six (6) times on the other side

Shoulder internal rotators

Lie on your back with your legs 6 to 8 inches apart with toes towards the ceiling

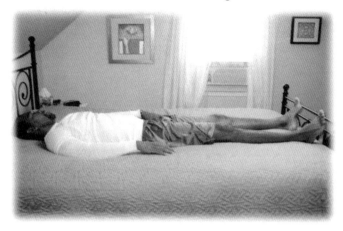

Raise your arms, shoulder level, palms facing your feet, with the upper part of your arm horizontal to your shoulders

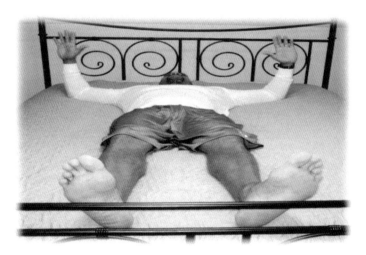

Bend your elbows while keeping the upper part of your arm pressed into the bed. Keep your forearms and hands are in front of your body

Rotate your forearms and hands up and back, extending as far as you can.

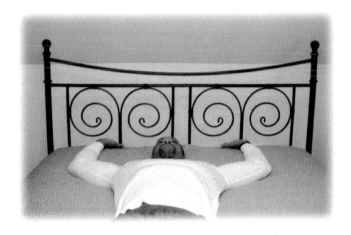

Hold for two (2) seconds

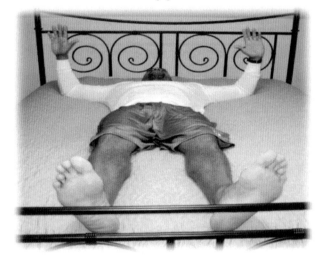

Repeat six (6) times

Shoulder external rotators

Lie on your back with your legs 6 to 8 inches apart with toes towards the ceiling

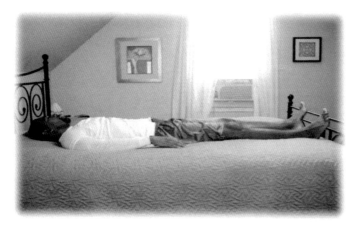

Raise your arms, shoulder level, palms facing your feet, with the upper part of your arm horizontal to your shoulders

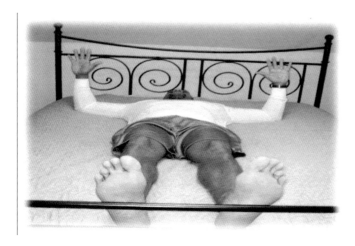

Bend your elbows while keeping the upper part of your arm pressed into the bed. Keep your forearms and hands are in front of your body

Rotate your forearms and hands down and back, extending as far as you can

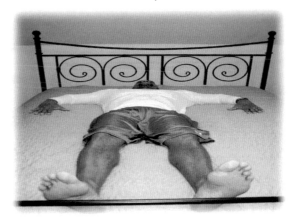

Hold for two (2) seconds

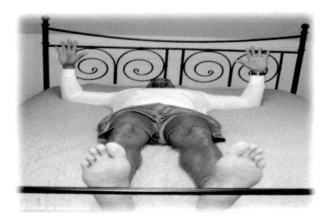

Repeat six (6) times

Forward elevation of the shoulder

Lie back with feet slightly apart and your arms at your side, and palm facing inwards

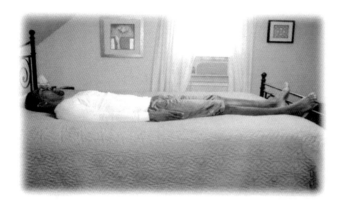

Raise one arm with your elbow locked, above your head

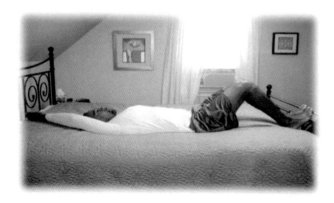

Press arm into bed and hold for 6 seconds
Repeat six (6) times

- Do the same exercise on the other side

Abdominal Pull

Lie flat on your back while resting your head on a pillow, with your knees up, if you can.

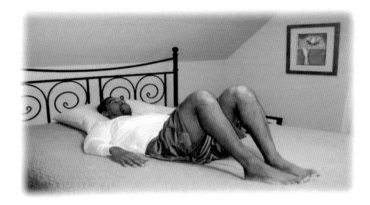

Make sure your lower back is pressed into the bed.

Gently pull your stomach (abdominal) muscles in, until the small of your back is flat against the bed. Hold this pose for 6 seconds, remembering to breathe while doing it.

While breathing out lift your head about 1 to 2 inches off the pillow.

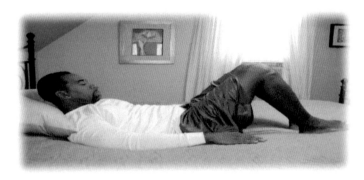

See if you can feel your abdominal muscles tighten.

Repeat six (6) times.

Pelvic tilt with Leg Extension

Lie in bed with your knees up

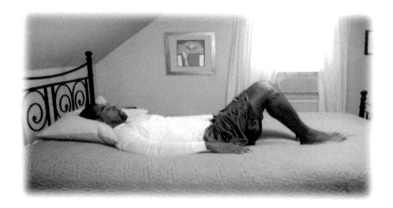

Gently kick out one leg as straight as you can.

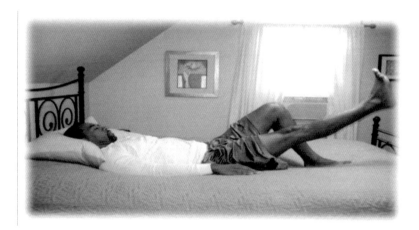

Hold for 6 seconds and then return to the original position.

Repeat six (6) times and then switch leg.

Additionally, you can bring both legs up to your chest, hold for six (6) seconds. This will stretch out the lower back.

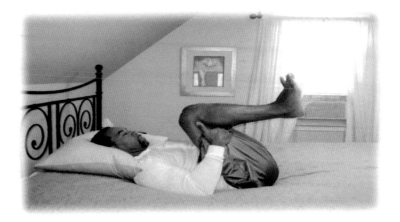

Lower your legs down to the bed.

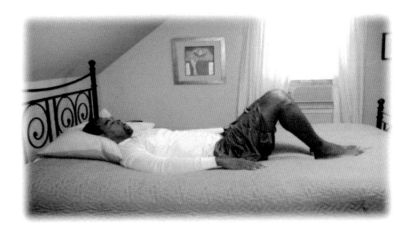

Repeat this stretch six (6) times

Arm Exercises

Lie in bed with your arms stretched above your head; squeeze the shoulder blades together while pressing your arms into the bed.

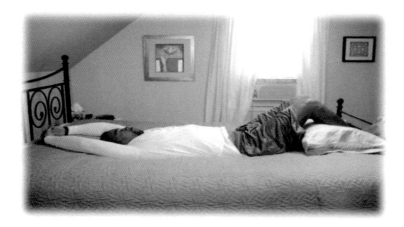

Hold for 6 seconds and release, with your arms back to your sides, hunch your shoulders up to your ears and hold for 6 seconds.

Release them slowly and lower your arms to your sides with palms facing in

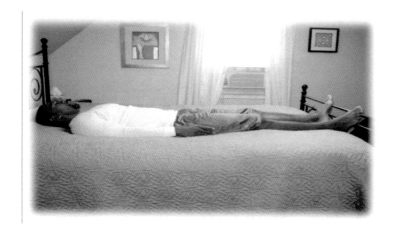

Repeat eight (8) times.

Quadriceps Exercises

Sit up in bed with your back as straight as possible. Place a pillow under your legs with legs straight out in front of you.

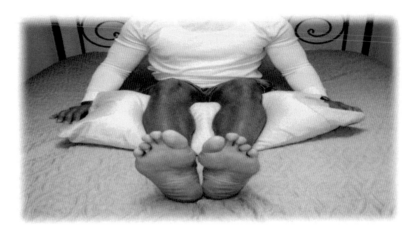

Keeping your toes pointed toward the ceiling and focus on pressing the backs of your legs down into the pillow.

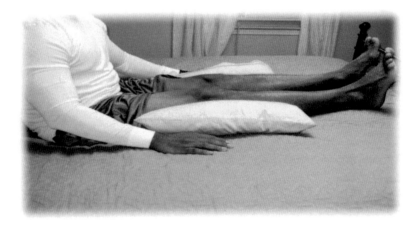

You may want to place your hands on your thighs so you can feel those muscles working.

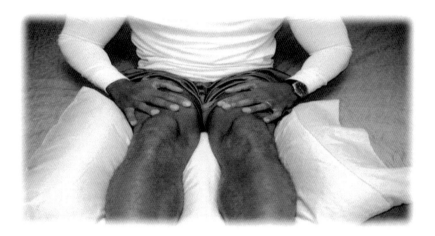

For a more advanced workout,

Lie in bed with one knee bent by placing the foot of the same leg flat on the bed while, keeping your other leg extended

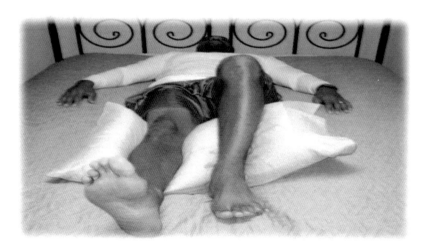

Lift the foot of your bent leg off the bed

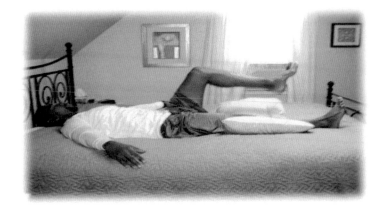

Extend your leg.

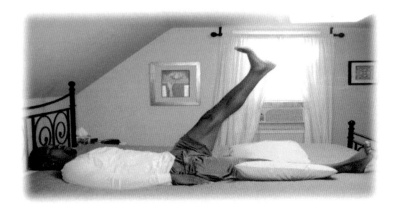

Bend and extend that leg ten (10) times

Repeat this exercise six (6) times

Repeat movement with other leg.

Gluteal and Hip Exercises

Lie flat on your back with your legs bent

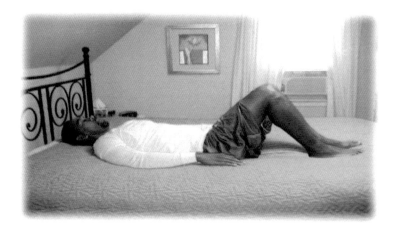

Press your feet into the bed, tighten your buttocks and lift your buttocks off the bed.

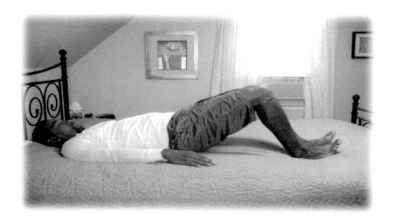

Hold the contraction for 15 seconds, then release.

Repeat six (6) times.

Lower back and back of legs stretch

Lie flat on your back while resting your head on a pillow, with your legs straight.

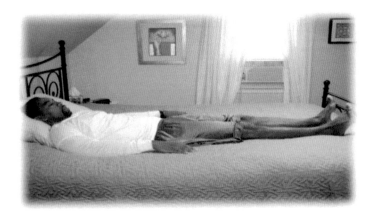

Bend your knees and pull your legs in towards chest to stretch the lower back and the back of your legs

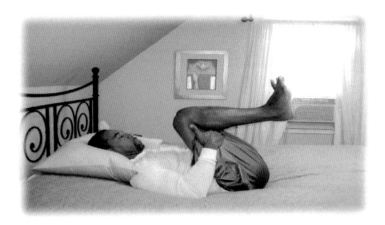

Repeat this stretch six (6) times

Hip Strengtheners

Lie on your right side in bed with head on a pillow, and right arm under your head.

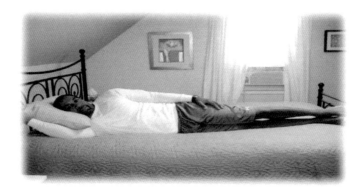

Bend your knees and gently press your ankles together. Place a pillow between your legs.

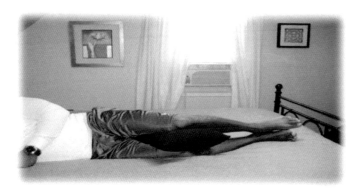

Tighten your stomach muscles and squeeze your knees together as tightly as possible. **Hold this tension for 8 seconds.**

Release the tension and return to the original position.

Relax for 10 seconds.

Repeat six (6) times.

Thigh Squeezers

Lie flat on your back while resting your head on a pillow, with your knees up.

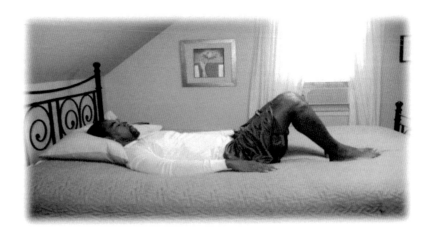

Place a pillow between your knees.

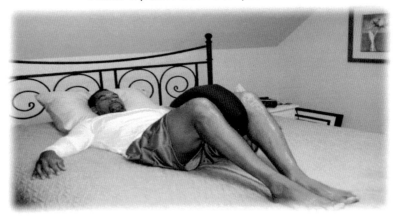

Press your thighs together and squeeze the pillow.

Hold this tension for eight (8) seconds.

Release the tension and relax for 10 seconds.

Repeat six (6) times.

Air Pedaling

Lie flat on your back with a pillow under your head while keep your arms at your sides and pressed against the bed.

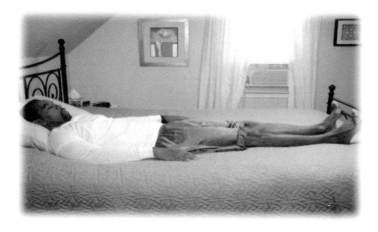

Lift both legs, bending at the knees.

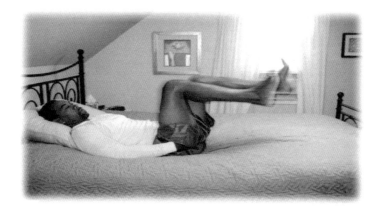

Pull the knees in toward your chest.

Begin the exercise by mimicking a bicycle pedaling motion.

Extend one leg out and rotate it in a circular motion.

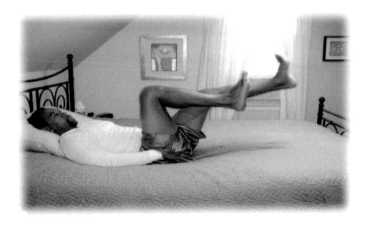

As the knee comes back toward your chest, extend the other leg and perform the same motion.

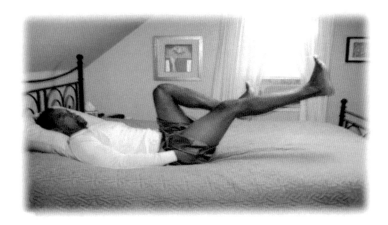

Perform the air pedaling movement for 20 seconds.

Rest for 20 seconds

Repeat six (6) times.

Leg Kicks

Lie flat on your back with a pillow under your head while keeping your arms at your sides and pressed into the bed.

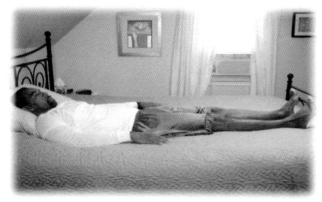

Raise your left leg and bend at the knee

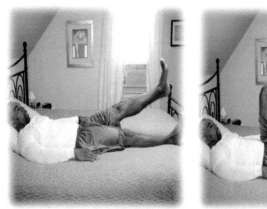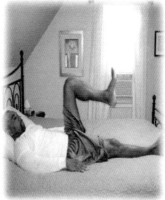

Pull the knee in toward your chest slowly and inhale.

Extend the leg outward keeping it elevated and exhale.

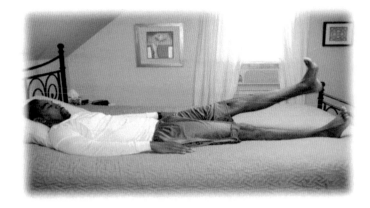

Repeat 10 times, and then switch legs.

Repeat six (6) times

Pull your legs in towards chest to stretch the lower back and the back of your legs

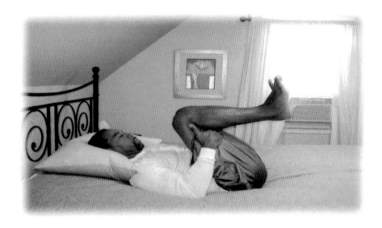

Hold stretch for 10 seconds

Repeat six (6) times.

Leg Curls

Lie on your stomach with a pillow under your head and arms resting under the pillow. Extend your legs straight back.

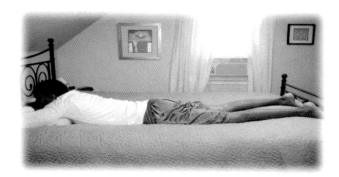

Slowly curl your legs toward your buttocks while exhaling.

Curl your leg as far as you can, contract the back of your legs.

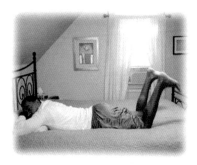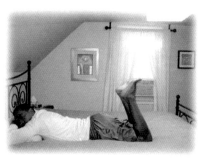

Squeeze for two (2) seconds

Slowly return your leg to the starting position and inhale.

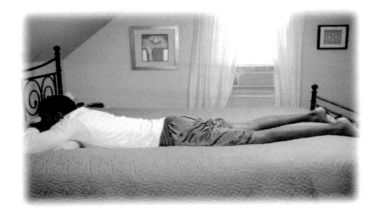

Repeat eight (8) times

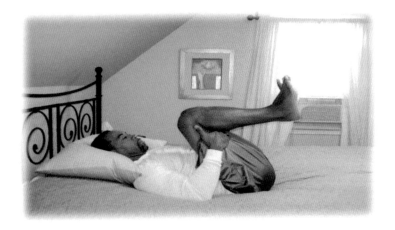

Return onto your back and stretch

Hold stretch for 10 seconds

Repeat six (6) times.

Leg Lifts

Lie flat on your back while resting your head on a pillow with legs extended straight.

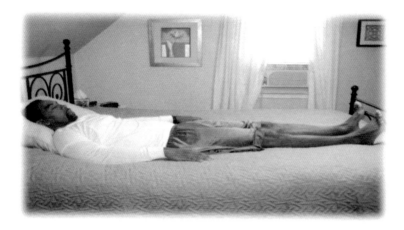

Slowly raise your right leg without bending at the knee.

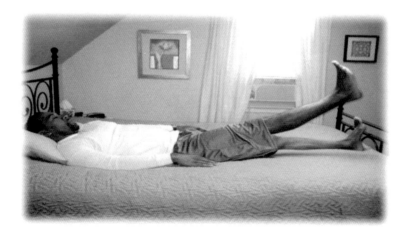

Raise the leg until it is perfectly vertical if you can.

Hold for 10 count at the top of the movement

Then slowly return the leg to its starting position as you inhale.

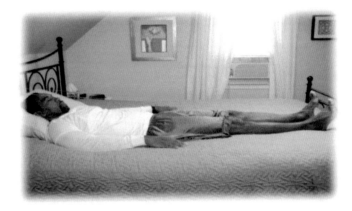

Repeat eight (8) times,

Switch sides

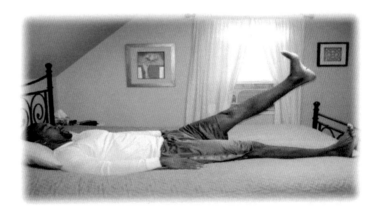

Do two to three sets total.

Keep your hands at your side to help stabilize and balance yourself.

Superman

Lie facedown on your pillow, legs straight and slightly apart with hands under your pillow as pictured

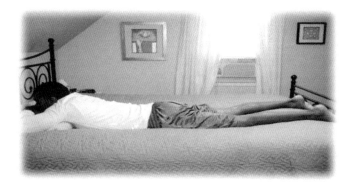

While keeping legs straight lift your legs as high as you can off the bed while exhaling.

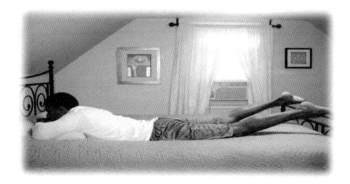

Look down at the bed and relax your neck and head throughout **the exercise.**

Stop when you feel a slight tension in your lower back.

Hold this position for five (5) seconds and then lower your legs onto the bed.

Repeat six (6) times

15010635R00017

Made in the USA
Charleston, SC
12 October 2012